Alzheimer's:
The Person Within

Alzheimer's:
The Person Within

a new pathway to joyful and fulfilling interaction with the memory impaired

Linda Marie Hemm

Writers Club Press
New York Lincoln Shanghai

Alzheimer's: The Person Within
a new pathway to joyful and fulfilling interaction with the memory impaired

Writers Club Press
an imprint of iUniverse, Inc.

For information address:
iUniverse
2021 Pine Lake Road, Suite 100
Lincoln, NE 68512
www.iuniverse.com

ISBN: 0-595-25748-8

Printed in the United States of America

I dedicate this book to the many dementia patients I worked with over the years, for they were my teachers.

Contents

Foreword

Some people seem to be born with a gift when it comes to caring for others. Linda Hemm is one of those people. Her genuine concern for the understanding and treatment of those suffering from Alzheimer's disease or any age related dementia is evidenced by the creation of this book.

Her knowledge comes from years of hands on experience both in-home health care and in private residential facilities. She continues working in this field with its joys and sorrows because she is following her heart.

As her co-worker, I observed Linda first hand. I have always admired her ability to relate to the elderly, especially those who need special care and understanding.

I have learned much from her and feel that there is a great need for the information Linda has provided in this book.

Sally Bartlett: NA, RCP

             *   *   *

There are those vocations which require, or, at the least, are more successfully pursued with an academic education. Linda's career is not one of those. During the years I have spent with her and the countless hours of assisting her in the editing process I have come to realize that hers is a field to which no formal degrees apply. I have learned that it takes a special gift of genuine care, sensitivity, compassion, and a lot of knowledge gained from experience to understand and to have meaningful interaction with persons afflicted by mental degeneration.

My brother, sisters, and I feel very fortunate in that we, at the time of this writing, have the opportunity to benefit from Linda's knowledge in learning to understand and better interact with our own dementia stricken mother. This insight has at times made the difference between frustrated despair and understanding compassion. Via her writing, I am very proud to know that others may also benefit in the same way.

Gordon E Hoffman: husband of the author

Acknowledgements

For me, it is one thing to have important information and the desire to share it with others. It is quite another to put it on paper and arrange it into proper form and readable text. For helping me to accomplish that, and for their constant support and much appreciated critique, I am so thankful to:

My husband, G. Edward Hoffman

My good friends

    Sally Bartlett

    Kathy Holmquist

My sister-in-law, Marlene Benson

Introduction

Information now available can help us to have a better understanding of the dementia process from a medical standpoint. Of course, we all hope that research will someday teach us possible prevention techniques. But, until preventive measures become effective, many, if not most of us, will experience the symptoms of progressive mental deterioration in a mother, father, grandparent, spouse, or other loved one. Therefore, it becomes imperative that we gain a better understanding of how to confront these symptoms and to learn, as much as possible, ways to break through the barriers that those symptoms present. Only by doing this can we preserve the dignity of the victim and, at the same time, provide for peace in our own lives.

This handbook is designed for the family member because that is where I saw the largest audience and therefore the greatest need. However, it is of no less value as a tool for the clinician. It is designed to offer specific instructions on interaction techniques that can help you, the daughter, son, spouse, friend, or professional caregiver, to maintain stimulating mental and physical activity in the life of the afflicted person.

I have deliberately kept the chapters in this manual short and to-the-point in order to make the information readable and understandable for everyone. You will find no wordy theories or lengthy discourse, only sound advice that I learned and have used successfully over and over again.

There are many types of age related dementia, including that which is commonly diagnosed as resulting from Alzheimer's disease. Most of the time we cannot know for certain what is the exact underlying cause. Therefore, I have also used the terms "dementia" and "memory impaired" to cover all forms.

CHAPTER ONE

Discovering the Joy of the Moment

The things that I have learned and continue to learn every day as a caregiver are too important to keep to myself. That is because there is still a person inside each cloak of dementia—a person capable of joy, sadness, laughter, tears, love, fear, and loneliness. There is a person in there whose needs can be tended to, but, only if we know how. It has been my quest, hopefully it is also yours, to learn how to provide as much joy for this person and to remove as much fear and confusion as we have the ability to do so.

Care giving has been a wonderfully rewarding experience for me. There is always a lot of joy to be found in providing pleasant moments for those who are incapable of providing their own. I understand that we are all individuals, and very different from each other. I realize that, for some, being a caregiver in the intimate, hands-on, sense, comes almost naturally, I am one of those. For others it will be a learning process born out of necessity. And for some it may even be an uncomfortable, if not impossible role. So, no guilt trips, please. We are all endowed with different talents and abilities, and, when the need arises there is a valuable role in which each person can make a positive contribution to the care of a dementia afflicted loved one. Whatever the extent of your personal involvement, the objective must be to make every occasion a purposeful, valuable, and, hopefully joyful time both for the indisposed and for you. In order to do that, each family member, even if you will only be an occasional visitor, needs to have an understanding of the dementia process. Why? There are at least three important reasons:

1) So that you will know how to interact in ways that minimize the possibility for negative responses and maximize the opportunity to experience happy results.

2) The persons who are involved as daily caregivers need all of the support, encouragement and intelligent help that they can get. When dealing directly with a memory impaired person on a frequent basis it may become very draining to the extent that the caregiver can easily lose some ability to cope. You can be there for them only if you know how.

3) You will, by learning and utilizing the information within these pages, gain much insight and, thereby, a new appreciation, not only for the dementia process but for life itself. This is knowledge that can be invaluable now and useful during the remainder of your life time.

I believe it is important that those who are now or will be providing care understand that effective care giving is a learning process. As I have already suggested, for some it comes easier than for others. There will be some frustrating times, but each experience is a part of a process that will create a stronger, more empathetic, insightful, and, certainly, a more fulfilled, YOU.

I can say these things with confidence because I have been there. Having over eleven years as an Activity Director for an Alzheimer facility and in home care for dementia patients, I can share with you the specifics of my own hands on experience. I have danced the dances and sung the songs with these people. We have cried together and laughed till we were giddy. We have gardened, set tables, shared parties, and enjoyed the

moments together. The experiences I share with you are about understanding the value of empathy and respect. They are about dignity and
caring; about walking hand in hand down an unfamiliar path together;
about cherishing each moment we've been given. They are about understanding, creating and treasuring the joy of the moment.

Perhaps I am more emotional than some, but, I am not ashamed to say
that my first years of facility work were, sometimes, accompanied by many
tears. On a good note these were seldom tears of sadness but, rather, from
seeing the positive difference I could make in someone's life. They were
from all the joy-filled moments we were able to have together. Small
things can make a big difference in the daily life of a person held captive
by dementia. You can make that difference when you learn how to create
these special moments. As you learn these techniques and begin to put
them to use, I encourage you to keep a journal of what I call, joy notes. I
do this with many of my clients and it provides me with incredible memories that I can also share with the patient's family. I have created a section
at the end of this book for you to record your special moments. It is enti-
tled *Joy Notes*.

When a diagnosis of dementia is made, know this: life is not over.
Changes will occur; they always do. And with those changes, comes the
challenge of coping with them. The success that I have experienced as I
accumulated and utilized these techniques in my interactions is proof positive that the quality of life for the victim can be significantly enhanced. At
the same time, our own frustration may be significantly reduced. I found
that the fulfillment I experienced during these times of sharing life with
the patients was therapy, not only for them, but also for me.

So, as you read this booklet and go about caring for your memory
impaired patient and/or loved one, always keep these important points in
mind:

1) Even though you may not be comfortable in a "caregiver" role,
   there is an extremely valuable purpose that you can fulfill.

2) Becoming an effective caregiver is a learning process that can offer many rewards.

3) It is the small things that can make a big difference to the person with diminished capacity.

4) You must focus on the now—not yesterday or tomorrow—in learning how to create the joy of the moment.

5) Discovering the joy of the moment is the key to creating happy and rewarding interaction with those who are memory impaired.

CHAPTER TWO

Our Verbal Interaction

Before Alzheimer's disease struck, David had been a very successful engineer, world traveler, husband, father and grandfather. At the time of the following occurrence, David was 81 years old and in his third year as a resident in our Alzheimer's facility. It was the Holiday season and our residents and family members were gathering for a few hours of food and activities. During the pre dinner activities I noticed that David had pulled his chair into a far corner of the dining room. He was completely overwhelmed by the barrage of conversation and other noisy commotion. He was confused and angry, and had withdrawn into himself to escape what he could not handle. His own family, without realizing it, was making matters worse by trying to reason with him, not understanding his special needs.

Talking is a part of almost all interaction and should be approached with much care. David's stressful situation could have been avoided if his family had understood and used communication methods geared to his state of mind. When dealing with dementia, first impressions are very important because once stress begins to build it is difficult to undo. Even though David's was a social situation the same basic rules apply anytime verbal communications are initiated.

Whether you are talking to your closest relative or some one you barely know, your approach should always be very simple and direct. Begin by making eye contact and introducing yourself. Even though you may already know the person well, their diminished capacity dulls the ability to recall so that the introduction may be needed by way of reminder. David's confusion may well have been in part because he did not fully recognize his family members. It is important to speak very slowly with deliberate pronunciation, but in a soothing mid-tone, and to use short sentences that are broken up into a few words at a time.

For example: "Hello, my name is Helen," will become, "**H e l l o** (pause) **My n a m e** (pause) **Is H e l e n.**"

Consistency is very important so try to use the same speaking pattern throughout your communicative efforts. Always keep in mind that speaking loud and fast can confuse thought patterns and stimulate agitation thereby precluding the very opportunity for positive communications. In this case, several family members were trying to talk to David in the same conversation causing him to experience confusion and the resulting need to withdraw from everyone.

David's reaction, by this time, was anger such that he tried to push a family member away. This was the only thing his mind knew to do to get away from what was stressing him. Sometimes, when the indisposed becomes obstinate and makes a negative gesture it is easy to get our own feelings hurt. Therefore, it is ultra important to know and continuously remind yourself of this truth: As dementia advances so goes the ability to think rationally. You are the one who is able to reason. If a negative reaction does occur do not take it personally and, by all means, do not give up. You are needed. Learning exactly what will work in your situation is a process that takes time to perfect. If you are willing to believe that a real and valuable person still exists behind that barrier, then you will succeed and your patience and forbearance will be wonderfully rewarded by a positive response.

Speak slowly, use short sentences, and always look directly into the eyes when speaking. Too soft may be hard to hear but too loud may cause confusion. Unless your loved one is hard of hearing, moderation is the word. In social situations, shield the indisposed from stressful commotion and indulge their attention in quiet words or sensory stimuli such as we will be discussing in further chapters.

* * *

Ruth Wilson, 84 years old, was one of my in-home dementia care patients for only a short time. One morning when I arrived at the Wilson's home to begin my shift Ruth was literally having a tantrum; throwing things around including her clothes, crying, and refusing to bathe. I managed to calm her down after some time but did not learn until later what was causing these outbreaks of childlike anger. Upon a subsequent visit I arrived early and realized that the caregiver whom I was replacing, though otherwise a wonderful, caring person, had been talking down to Ruth as though she were a child—correcting her, telling Ruth how to do things in her own kitchen, etc.

Even though Ruth had become childlike in many of her actions, in her own mind she is still mother, wife, woman. Her need was to be treated as such. This care giver had not yet learned that retention of the need for independence and role respect remains very strong in many dementia patients.

I have seen the same reaction to similar treatment many times. It seems to be one of our first reactions to treat the child-like mother or father as a child. I can almost guarantee that if you do so, you had better be prepared to reap some very negative results. Regardless of the infantile actions we may observe, it is a must, from my observation, that we talk to mother and father with the same respect they expected pre-dementia because they continue to need that and they continue to need the same feeling of independence. The mother and father part is still alive in there. Please realize and learn that there are ways to give the feeling of independence and still maintain control. Is it a challenge?—yes. Is it worth the trouble?—you bet.

This chapter may be short on words, but, it is long on significance. These are some of the basic skills that you will need to take with you into all interactive engagements with your patient; more and more as the dementia progresses. The earlier you learn the skills the easier it will be later on:

1) Talking must be simple and direct using continuous eye contact.
2) If they are sitting, you sit. If standing, try to stand in front of them.
3) Speak in a soothing mid-tone and use short sentences.
4) Always be aware that there is a real person in there.
5) Dignity and independence are most valued possessions.
6) Simple things can make a big difference in their daily life.

Remember, positive interactive response begins with positive communications techniques. When planning and implementing verbal communication or any other form of interaction with a person who is afflicted with any type of dementia, your primary objective must be to make that moment in life a positive experience for that individual. You must learn what it takes to do that. Your subsequent objective, by accomplishing the first, will be to make that interaction a less stressful, more pleasant, and, even a rewarding process. You can do it!

CHAPTER THREE

Social Situations

Tori's birthday party was scheduled for 2:30pm. Her children had ordered their mother's favorite cake from the best bakery in town. As Tori's guests began to arrive I looked around and Tori had disappeared. When I found her she was sitting on a bench in the far corner of the indoor walkway. She was sobbing. I approached her slowly and spoke softly, bringing my body down to her level, and asked her why she was upset. With tears streaming down her face, she looked me in the eyes and said, "I'm afraid. I don't know who let in all those people, and, who are they?"

No one had spent the time necessary to prepare Tori for her birthday party and she had become frightened because she did not recognize her children and grandchildren. David's situation, in chapter one, was similar except that his reaction was one of anger.

Social situations involving the dementia patient are highly recommended and can result in a fulfilling family event. However, they also have the potential to be very uncomfortable and trying time for both the family and the indisposed. Because much of the fear and other discomfort experienced by a memory impaired person stems from confusion, it is absolutely imperative to eliminate the opportunity for confusion as much as possible. Here are three important steps:

The first is to educate the family members. Neither Tori's or David's families were aware of the need to identify themselves, nor were they informed as to the importance of communicating with their loved one in a slow, easy, one-at-a-time manner.

The second step is to prepare the patient with reminders of the event. Verbal reminders help but only if repeated frequently. The most effective are large signs such as: **TORI'S BIRTHDAY PARTY—or—DAVID'S THANKSGIVING DINNER**—placed where the patient can readily see and read them throughout the course of the event.

The third step is to maintain the identity process. You must always keep in mind that the memory impairment causes continuous lapses in memory and, therefore requires constant reminders. However, we know that repetitious verbal reminders can become irritating and are often even futile. The solution? Name tags. Simple, but it works—**NICE LARGE LETTERS THAT ARE EASY TO READ**. Depending on the progression of the dementia, it may be very important to include the relationship in order to aid in the identity process. For example:

HELEN
IS
DAVID'S DAUGHTER

David no longer has to deal with the frustrating confusion of trying to identify who this person is because he is reminded every time he sees the name tag, "My daughter, Helen."

In addition, the process of creating the name tag can be great fun and will help prepare the patient for the event. I found that most memory impaired persons still enjoy hearing the sound of their own name, so make it a big deal. First ask if you can print his/her name on a name tag and if you can place it on his/her person. Now, before you actually do the placing show it to him/her and ask if you have the name spelled correctly (even though you know that you did). These actions make the care receiver feel a part of what is going on. It also provides reassurance and a feeling of safety, that he/she is among family and friends. I cannot convey to you how many times I have seen a person with a down turned face lift his chin and smile when I said his name, thanked him for joining our group, and gave him a tag with his very own name on it. I experience my own tears of joy when I see small things like this make a very big difference in a person's every day struggle with dementia.

Include simple art clips on the name tag if possible, perhaps with a favorite animal, bird, or sport. This is almost always a big hit. Seasonal changes can be followed. For example, use pumpkins at Halloween or Christmas trees at Christmas time. Any clip art used must be positive. Never use black cats or frowning, frightening, pumpkins or witches. Please note that I have suggested printing, rather than writing on the name tags. Try always to use simple and concise print; large print and black ink are easier for most to read. White or pastel paper works best.

Use name tags at any and all social functions where interaction will be taking place, even family gatherings large or small. You may think dad would certainly recognize his sister, or grandchild, and, even if he does now that is most certain to change as the impairment progresses. Certainly, it is not worth taking the chance of dad being upset. Remember, it is much more pleasant and, believe me, a lot easier to prevent a negative situation than to turn it around once it happens. Doing these things can help make social situations easy and comfortable for every one; less tension and stress leaves more room for smiles and other positive interaction.

You will find more helps that will relate to social situations in the following chapters. Just remember to reduce the opportunity for frustration by eliminating any cause for frustration:

1) Increase your own awareness and find ways to educate other family members as to the special needs of the memory impaired.

2) Prepare your care receiver for any social event through repetitive telling about the occasion, and what family members will be there.
3) Use signs to identify the event for the patient.
4) Name tags, name tags, name tags.

CHAPTER FOUR

Validation

Lacy, 83 years old lived at home with her husband, Bob. She was exhibiting fits of anger, in general being obstinate, and, typical of many dementia patients, she didn't think she needed a bath.

Their first caregiver was a daughter, Gail. Though she loved her mother very much, she became so confused and frustrated with Lacy's behavior that she felt she could no longer fill that position. Enter, yours truly.

It was imperative that I become intimately aware of the nature of the negative interactions between Gail and her mother. Next I needed to find ways to establish a positive relationship with Lacy so that I could determine the underlying reasons for her undesirable conduct. Through patient, calm, slow questioning, and pleasant conversation I first learned what Lacy liked (I try to stay away from does not like questions). She loved music so we sang songs together and I validated her by praising her on having a wonderful voice. She liked to share hugs so I validated that by sharing hugs with her. She also reminisced that she liked to take her bath at night and, then put on her robe because "it always feels so good". Then I knew: Lacy's reluctance to bathe came about for two reasons. She had forgotten the good feeling it gave her (being clean is no longer a good enough reason to take a bath); and secondly her long time daily routine had been upset. Because it fit better into her daily care giving schedule, Gail had been trying to make her take a bath in the morning.

Because my first challenge was to get Lacy to take her bath every day, I had to validate her expressed feeling for the warm bath at night and then reinforce that by making it happen. It was not without a couple initial fits of temper that Lacy reluctantly stepped into the tub. But once she experienced that warm bubbly water along with a nice back massage and then her warm cuddly robe, the problem was over. In fact, Lacy began to look forward to her bath time and would often talk about it during the day.

Lacy's demeanor almost instantly made a big change for the better. I learned that she was a very agile lady who loved music and dancing. So when she opened the door for me each morning I would began singing a song. She would join in and then I would give her a big hug and tell her how glad I was to hear her beautiful voice. She would always tell me how glad she was that I was there because she could have so much fun with me. No, it doesn't always go this well, and, yes, it may even go better, but I have yet to experience continued negative results when I consistently apply this type of effort. In any event, my goal is that you can see the enormous value of, first LEARNING, then, VALIDATING the activities, needs, and routines that are important to the person you are caring for.

As I use the term validate, it means to acknowledge and show support for a person's expressed need or desire. That also infers my acceptance of the person's state of mind, whatever that may be, so that I can allow that person his or her dignity.

In today's world of psycho-babble one word that has become increasingly popular is, "enable". We have learned that if we don't show our disapproval of certain negative actions we will, in effect, enable, encourage, and empower the person to continue or even increase that activity. Unfortunately this is often a first reaction many of us may have to displays of anger, obstinacy, or reclusive behavior. Please don't go there.

These seeming acts of misconduct can in reality be the impaired mind's way of communicating an emotional or physical distress. To punish that act of communication can serve to frustrate the situation further and even close off any chance for positive interaction. Rather than becoming disgruntled and/or forceful, which can only cause further agitation; you must be willing to react to the behavior in an effectual manner. The way to begin that process is to reach out with all of your patience to find the reasons for the behavior.

For me interaction with the mentally impaired can be a genuine source of joy. It is almost always a challenge that I am eager to win. It is so rewarding because I get to see the joy of the moment over and over again. Maybe I look at it a little like I did my mothering days in that I seldom tired of finding a way to change my baby's wailing cries of unhappiness into a grin or a giggle. That was a continuous repetitive effort born of love, need, and caring.

Sometimes even negative conduct can be validated for positive results. One patient, Ruth, had been experiencing paranoia. During these times she became very distraught and would accuse a son or daughter of stealing from her. It is only natural to defend ones self and so the siblings constantly denied any such doing. Of course, Ruth knew they were lying which only made her more upset.

After learning the need for validation, an accused daughter, Ann, no longer tried to deny the theft. Rather, she simply answered the accusation, "OK, mom, I'll bring it back".

That was it. It was over. No hassle. Mom felt better and now could forget the whole thing. Ann might even get a little chuckle out of her righteous deceit, especially knowing that it had eliminated the usual, hurtful feelings on both sides. Yes, I said righteous deceit and that is exactly what it is. The only moral question in all of this is whether or not we harm the one we love. Ruth is not living in, or reacting to, reality when this paranoia is present. Therefore, all the reality in the world cannot solve the problem for her—it will, in fact, make matters worse. Sometimes we have to fight fire with fire and sometimes, I have learned, we have to fight unreality with unreality.

The more you get involved with your afflicted loved one or patient, the more creative you may become in finding ways to validate them which can in turn, stimulate increased activity. For example, you may allow and encourage simple tasks. You will need to experiment to know what tasks the individual can safely and successfully perform. If he or she is residing in your home or in a home under your supervision, you could include that person in daily living tasks like setting the table, sweeping the floor, folding clothes, dusting and vacuuming. Remember that these kinds of tasks must be limited to the person's abilities. Since each case is different, only by experimenting will you know those limits.

Ask for their help. Include your care receiver in small decision making, and give choices. For Example: "Should we use the red or yellow table-cloth?" Which of these two plates look best on this table? Keep the selection simple, perhaps between two objects. If the person cannot choose, make a selection yourself then ask if that choice is OK. You will no doubt get agreement.

And, then, VALIDATE—give rewards. Set your care recipient up for "wins and success." Their self-esteem is very fragile—you may tell your dementia loved one "thank you" or "good job" many times in one day and then repeat it all over again the next day. It may become necessary to reassure that person almost constantly. If this is what it takes, you must be prepared to do so.

It is extremely important to play along with the moment. As with all dementia reactions, do not try to reason. It accomplishes nothing positive and may well serve to frustrate your time together.

As I have stated before; with the loss of short term memory many things will need to be repeated. Try to accept that fact and simply go with it because there is no way for you to change it. You may find that there is a lot of peace to be found within ACCEPTANCE.

1) Determine the needs, wants and comfort zones of the patient.
2) Realize that you probably can't change these things. Unless it is a harmful behavior, it is usually best to go along.

3) Understand that validation is one of your most valuable tools. It can be used to reinforce a positive behavior, and also to release a negative thought pattern (think about that one).

4) Self-esteem can be very fragile, bolster it as often as you have opportunity.

CHAPTER FIVE

Reliving the Past

When I think of the significant role that a patient's past can play, I often think of Karen. Karen called each of her female caregivers, Carol. We just accepted that, not knowing the reason. Finally, in discussing this with a family member, we learned the reason. It turned out that Karen had had a very dear friend in her past. Carol was Karen's best friend in the second grade. Their friendship was so meaningful to her that later on, in her dementia, all females who were close to her became Carol.

An understanding of the care receiver's past history, with their various likes, dislikes, and pleasures can be immensely helpful in planning a more effective program of interaction. If you are caring for a close relative you will, no doubt, have this knowledge. If not, accumulate as much knowledge of his/her personal memorabilia as you can. As the memory impairment progresses Alzheimer patients remember much more about the long ago past, even their childhood, than they may recall about what happened in later years or even what happened minutes ago. Therefore, I found much greater basis for successful intercourse when I learned how to bring back memories from the past. Did the person enjoy reading, walking, crafts, games, sports? What were their early childhood years like—farm life, city life, etc.? Place of birth, and to whom? What about school days? How about working for a living? Did he hammer nails and saw wood? Did she teach grammar school?

When memorabilia plays a major part in your conversation, response will become much more lively, open, and meaningful, sometimes producing incredible stories from the past.

Knowledge of the role the past plays will also help you a lot in understanding the person's actions. For example, advanced patients often begin talking about going back home, sometimes even packing up their belongings. You will naturally think they are referring to the home where they last lived when in reality they are yearning for their childhood home. My mother-in-law frequently talks about her longing to go home. We know by asking her questions about the home that she is meaning the farm she grew up on in the prairies of Canada.

A thought to share: caregivers who make it a practice to compile notes of these reminisces can share these times with (other) family members. This can provide invaluable memories for them to keep and share for years after their loved one has gone.

*   *   *

Doris was fairly advanced in her dementia; having been very fashion conscious in the past, she still maintained great pride in her appearance. Once, while I was doing her hair and nails, she asked for the hand mirror. When she looked at her face she said, "That's not me". "Who is that?"

Loss of self identity is a common symptom of dementia. By using memorabilia from the person's past you will be able to place helpful reminders of their identity around them. For example: put a bulletin board up in the patient's bedroom using photos of family. Old photos of their earlier years are most valuable—the earlier the better. Clearly and boldly label each photo so that anyone who is visiting can read the caption aloud. Then encourage everyone who enters the person's room to look at the board and to read it, making sure the patient can hear. In general, try to make a big deal out of the photos. This board can become an instant communication tool for anyone entering the room. Everyone can benefit from it. Use it a lot.

Another invaluable item can be a small photo book that the care receiver can carry in a pocket or purse. Put his/her name and address in or on the front of the book. Again, be certain that each photo is captioned and easy to read. Having this book can make going to a social event or a day-care setting much more pleasant. It will no doubt become a prized possession, a center for interaction with others, and a way for the dementia person to simply pass time reminiscing. You will probably find yourself going through this book with your patient over and over, at their insistence. Very important: never remind your care receiver that you have already seen the book. Each time you must appear as though you had not seen the book before and are delighted that she/he can show it to you.

I sometimes consider working with dementia like acting on stage. Just like the stage, you may need to repeat a scene over and over until it is perfected and satisfies everyone. Then repeat it some more as needed. Remember, it is repetition only to you. To the afflicted mind it is a beautiful memory or thought process, fresh each time.

For some victims of dementia, work was their life and they were on the go all of their waking moments. All of their life has been spent in pursuit of life's many projects and/or pleasures. For these persons, though their abilities have diminished, the old habits don't necessarily go away. One of the demented ladies I cared for had made her career as a schedule manager, first for a governor, and later for a senator. During her days at the Alzheimer unit she diligently attended all of our committee meetings. I have found that many of these career types retain the need to be doing something or trying to help someone all the time. To be given that opportunity helps them to feel alive and valuable.

Keep in mind that this is a learning experience and as such it may take a little time for you to become comfortable. It will work if you are willing to go for it. The positive response is your reward and makes it all worth while. Remember:

1) The role that the past will play increases with progression of the dementia.
2) Understanding that role will help you to find positive ways to interact through reminiscing and the use of memorabilia.

CHAPTER SIX

Pet Therapy

In many cases animals can be very therapeutic for comfort and stimulation, whether as pets or observed in the wild. Of course, there are persons who have an aversion to a certain animal, or, maybe even animals in general. However, most enjoy touching animals or just watching them. Did the person like animals and have pets like dogs and cats? Were they raised on a farm? Do your homework. Try to find out this information if you do not already know it. With this information in hand, try to find someone with a dog to visit in your home or facility. In a city, most animal shelters have a list of people who enjoy sharing their dogs. Look for a dog that is calm in nature and does not move fast. Size is not that important and can be a personal preference. The dog should be clean and loving and kept on a leash or in hand during their visit. Cats can be included here, but are much harder to locate. They do not appreciate being moved around from place to place, and few accept strangers as dogs do.

If your loved one resides in a facility, the activity director may have opportunities to provide animal related settings. Some Zoos offer a mobile petting zoo and arrangements can be made for a visit. In my first two weeks of facility activity work, I received a phone call late on a Friday that the mobile Zoo was scheduled for a visit on the next day. I was not sure what to expect, but, I vividly remember that I and several of our dementia victims almost passed out when the Zoo volunteers lifted Inky, the black snake, out of his box! None of us wanted to hold him, but it was so much fun to watch the lively responses. I had to ask them not to bring Inky back—a little too much stimulus. The chickens, believe it or not, were the big hit of the day, and all told, the show was a great success.

Farm days are always a lot of fun. Owners are usually very generous about bringing their trained pot-bellied pig to come in and do tricks. Although the last one I saw probably would not be so generous next time. I arrived at the care center just as the pig's owners were walking him (her?) out to put him in the car. When I left several hours later every one was still outside sitting on the grass. That 300 pound pig absolutely refused to get into the car. I never did find out when or how they ever got that animal home. Watch for the reactions of your patient(s) during these programs. The possibilities are endless when it comes to animals—the joy and communication they can bring out of a human being.

I own a horse that I have used often for pet therapy. Though I can't bring him to the care facility, I love to talk about him and share my experiences. I try to make that a daily occurrence. Sueño (pronounced Swaynyo) is a real character and the patients loved to hear about his antics. One of the ladies actually memorized his name, which was quite remarkable, and made a point each day to ask me how "Sueño" was doing. One lovely spring day I got permission from her family and took her to meet Sueño. He was as entertaining as usual. As she stroked Sueño's face, she turned to me and shared an early memory experience from her childhood. She told of how she used to love to go to a place called Jantzen Beach, on the Columbia River near Portland, Oregon, to rent horses. She loved to feel the wind in her face and feel the horse galloping underneath her. It was so rewarding to see the joy that this experience brought to her. I recorded that story for the family who had not heard about that part of their mom's past.

Another favorite memory involves Kathy, a very dedicated daughter. Her mother, Betty, resided in the Alzheimer facility where I was on staff. One spring day Kathy brought in a batch of baby ducks. The residents had such a positive reaction that I went out and bought a plastic wading pool so that each time Kathy brought the ducks we could watch them swim. The residents really enjoyed this and it was fun for me to watch Kathy work through the challenges of transporting the ducks as they became bigger and bigger. Most of all, it was a joy to see the love connection between Kathy and her mother during these times.

Providing a bird watching area is a positive visual for all people. The birds will move in when you provide feed, water and housing. Try to include your care receiver in the feeding of the birds in any way possible.

Randy had lived his life as a very successful airplane engineer. He had two lovely daughters who adored him. After he was placed in an Alzheimer facility, they made every effort to make his room comfortable. For Christmas one of his daughters bought a bird feeder to hang outside his bedroom window. The bird feeder became a part of his life. He was too fragile to go out to fill the feeder but whenever it was empty he would find one of the staff members and demand that the feeder be filled "Right now!" Everyone learned to drop what they were doing and feed the birds!

Aquariums that are well maintained and filled with different sizes of fish can be very soothing and relaxing to view. If you are not experienced with fish, go to an expert in the field. The cover to the tank will need to be secured so that it cannot be opened easily. The fish food should be kept high in a cupboard out of reach. The tank should remain in an area where it can be monitored for tampering. Be certain to use shatter proof glass.

CHAPTER SEVEN

The Changing Role of the Senses

Though each Alzheimer's case is unique, as brain function degenerates, so also do the functions of the body. Among these are the five senses. It is important to know which of these abilities the afflicted loved one is still capable of using and to what extent. To do this, you will have to make your own assessment based purely on observation. Actually, if you are paying attention, you will gain this insight fairly easily. It is also very helpful when you can include the assistance of other family members.

Obviously, we seldom use one sense without another being affected. However, I have created a separate subtitle for each of the senses for reference sake.

The Sense of Hearing

(and music therapy)

Hearing is usually the first sense to deteriorate. Until that happens, music can be utilized therapeutically and is a very valuable tool for interactive communications.

Music therapy can be a beautiful experience. There are wonderful musical selections for just about any situation. However, for the most part, music selected from the days of the dementia victim's youth will be the music they will recall and respond to. The music of some of the greats like Glenn Miller, Benny Goodman and Lawrence Welk are invaluable for current elderly dementia patients.

I cannot tell you what a certain musical chord will trigger in any individual, but it can be an interesting and even rewarding experience. For example, I witnessed one younger victim of dementia break into a ballet while listening to a certain Christmas cassette. We were able to engage this person in dance for several months afterwards.

A desire to dance often accompanies music and can also be very therapeutic. But you will need to know some personal history before you try to engage an elderly person in any rigorous physical activity. If he or she loved to waltz and you know that they can still safely ambulate, encourage that person to dance with you. You will, no doubt, need to lead.

Any swaying to the music is therapy for the soul. In facility settings there may be several couples who loved to dance. Provide the setting for them to feel comfortable in doing so. Prepare yourself because such a scene can bring tears to your eyes, and you may have the good fortune to see and experience the communication of love more pronounced than you have ever seen it before. More than once I have had wives of dementia victims come to me with tears in their eyes after being able to dance with their dear husbands once again. They had stopped dancing in public long ago because their loved ones actions had become unpredictable and would often cause embarrassment. In the privacy of the facility they were able to hold one another close again.

Singing some of the good old songs together has always been a very positive experience. Even if you think that you cannot carry a tune, do it anyway. Who cares? This is not a talent contest, believe me, if it was, I would have been in big trouble. If your loved one does not join in, and sometimes that happens, keep singing anyway. Encourage him/her to sing with you, and you will usually soon have a duo—or a chorus in the case of group care.

Sing songs like "You are my sunshine" and "Row, row your boat." Several of these old songs are printed out in the songs section of this book. These are the songs of their youth. When they were young, gathering around and joining a sing-a-long was one of the favorite forms of entertainment. I have even experienced success with people who had very limited hearing ability, or could no longer hear at all. Bringing that person into a group setting can be a positive experience for both the person and the caregiver.

Even if hearing is gone there are ways that you can usually convey the song you are singing by pointing out the words in the book as they are being sung. Watch for their recognition of the song and their ease as they realize that you are including them. You are sending the message that they are just as important as the other voices in the crowd. Keep in mind old favorites work best.

When using printed music always keep rooms as well lit as possible. It has been found that poor lighting can be a factor in causing confusion.

Never use a songbook with the musical notes in it. The notes can be very confusing for dementia patients. That is why you will find no notes in the songs and hymns sections that I have included as an important part of this book.

If the person you are caring for has a religious faith, use the hymn section of this book or keep a hymnal to sing with them. Very basic devotions can also be included. You will have greater success by getting into some form of a regular routine. Your dementia person may have a favorite song or hymn. If so, try to sing it together every day. I love being in the middle of a group of my dementia patients singing the good old hymns. The most meaningful hymn for these dear people seems to be "Jesus loves me." This song even received positive responses from those who declared no particular faith.

One of my very favorite memories of singing with groups of Alzheimer victims involves a sweet man who came in for day care. His name was Ed and he loved to join in with us when the entire group was singing. He would leave the facility singing and when he returned to us he was singing. Each morning Ed would sing a "Good Morning to You" solo. Everyone loved his visits. I think he was the first person in my life to sincerely greet me with, "Hello Friend."

If you can play an instrument like the guitar or piano, use your wonderful talent to make someone's day. Stimulating the senses of the dementia afflicted can be a very rewarding experience. If you, like me, are not blessed with such talent, search out someone who would be willing to come and play live music for the person or group of persons you are working with. One caution though, it is usually best to try to keep the performance short, probably no more than a half hour. The stimulation is great therapy but just keep in mind that some patients tire rapidly, both physically and emotionally.

We had the good fortune to have a very dedicated guitar player come twice a month to play for our residents. She always asked if anyone had any requests. Gertrude was 84 years old and was raised in the South. When the guitar player asked Gertrude what her favorite song was. Gertrude's response was "The Tennessee Waltz." This dear guitar player did not know the requested song but spent a couple of months learning it for Gertrude. As the song was played, Gertrude beamed with sheer happiness grinning from ear to ear. Afterwards, she got up from her chair, walked over to the guitar player and thanked her for playing her song. That can be quite a feat for an Alzheimer's patient. From that time on the guitar player always played Gertrude's song just for her. The sincere talent and old songs of our volunteer guitar player reached the hearts of everyone who listened. Both residents and staff looked forward to her visits. Seeing the smile on Gertrude's face made all of my efforts even more worthwhile.

Normally live music is not even an option; however, there are many good videos available. Musical instrumentals set to nature are usually a big hit. Other suggestions are tapes of children playing and singing and musical variety shows such as re-runs of Lawrence Welk. You can use these videos as music therapy, playing different tapes at different times of the day. There is an exception. Though we may be soothed by ocean scenes with sounds of the beach and the roar of the ocean, this is usually not well accepted by someone with dementia. It may well be just irritating noise to that person. Make your selections wisely and watch for a positive or negative reaction.

Many other sounds can also provide positive stimulation. I have successfully used cassettes or CD's that feature birds chirping to help my patient wake up and realize that it is morning. Another proven technique is to provide cricket sounds in the evening which can be reminiscent of sitting on the front porch at night before going to bed. If your care receiver can still hear these sounds, they can help cue the body as to what time of day it actually is. Maintaining the feeling for the time of day will be very important to both the caregiver and the patient.

NOTE: as a side benefit, I have found that keeping persons with dementia active enough during the daytime will usually bring about a more sound sleep at night.

The Sense of Smell

The loss of this sense often seems to be in a race with the loss of hearing. Work with this sense for as long as possible. The sense of smell can be valuable in bringing back old memories like mom's kitchen, the barn, the workshop, or the garden.

An active imagination will provide you with the scents required to stir up old memories. For example, cooking and baking can fill a place with good smells and bring back warm memories of the past.

My most positive success with smell stimulation has been to show an item, whether it be a cookie, cake, dead fish, or fresh flower and discuss the smell. This will usually lead the person into recalling a memory from the past and a story often ensues. If this should happen, try to record as much of the story as possible. Ask questions that will guide the person along the path of his or her memories. Again, you will, no doubt, hear additional stories from memories of childhood experiences.

This experience comes to my mind immediately. One of my male coworkers was an avid fisherman. One day, having caught a very large bass, he brought it in to show some of the residents. Two of the residents had loved fishing when young, and what a barrage of fishing memories that big bass stirred up. Their eyes lit up, their arms came to life and we all heard several stories about the one that got away. Certainly the stimulation here was as much sight as smell, but most stimulation will affect more than one sense. You do not have to be a fisherman to know that fish have a certain odor about them.

The bottom line is that there are a lot of smells around that can bring back to the dementia afflicted mind, vivid memories which may motivate positive response and a media for stimulus and interaction. Use them often.

The Sense of Speech

As dementia progresses, speech will become more and more difficult. It is an important exercise to involve your loved one in some form of speech pattern everyday. Make it part of your daily routine. A list of simple trivia such as asking, "You can lead a horse to water but..." (wait for the answer) "you can't make him drink." You will find this type of trivia in my book of games. This type of interaction is usually a huge success and you will want to use it as often as possible.

If your care receiver can still see well enough, try to get him or her to read out loud for you. If the words come out transposed simply ignore it. Even if a blunder becomes obvious, it can usually be a form of amusement for both of you.

Ask if your care receiver has heard any good jokes lately. The answer will usually be no. Then you should be prepared to tell one.

There is a cemetery nearby that I cannot drive past without having tears well up in my eyes. They are not tears of sadness but tears of joy that a very special man, Stan, brought to everyone on our staff. Stan was afflicted with Alzheimer's disease but had such a great sense of humor that he often made our day. I frequently put together theme days that I would simply call "shows". One of these was a rock show for which we asked staff and families of the residents to bring in any rocks or rock stories to share. One of our staff members brought in a rock from the 1970's called a "rock concert." It was a large flat rock with a bunch of small pebbles standing on end on top of the flat surface. Each of the small pebbles had been painted in bright colors and each one had a painted funny face. When I showed the rock to Stan, he reached out, held it in his hand and said "Watch this." He then cocked his head and made a face just like the character faces on the rock. Fortunately, I had my camera in hand and captured the moment on film. Stan taught me so much about the importance of being able to laugh at ourselves and share the funnybones with everyone around us.

No, we can't all be comedians no matter how hard we may try, but a little humor can go a long way in providing positive interactions with our impaired loved one. Regardless of how it is accomplished, the patient needs to be encouraged to vocalize. Humor is just one very positive way to do that. Sometimes it just happens. I don't remember jokes well, so I depend upon other written materials to aide me in my endeavors to create laughter. On one particular day I read a joke that I thought was very funny but got no response. So, I went on to another activity. All of a sudden one of the ladies began to giggle, then another, and another. Soon we all began to laugh until tears were running down our faces. I never did figure out what triggered our laughing session but it was wonderful therapy for all.

The Sense of Sight

Creating activities is much easier if the dementia person still has use of sight. However, those with impaired vision can usually see items and follow movement; it is just that smaller details will be more difficult for them to identify. For example, if roses are delivered and placed on a table, they may become lost in the background of the room. So it is often necessary to bring the flowers directly into the person's field of vision where his/her eyes can focus. Try to remember to do this with each visit because, each time you make the dementia person aware of the flowers it will be like the first time he/she has ever seen them. In other words, it is quite likely that there will be no recall of having seen the roses before so that the person will be delighted each time with the beauty of the roses and also with your efforts to please them. Apply this insight to anything that you wish to share with your impaired loved one. Never assume that the dementia person visually comprehends an object just because the object is in sight.

In later stages of dementia other items such as books, magazines and newspapers will need to be shown to the person just as the roses were. Never assume that the person is enjoying something just because you feel it is within their range of sight. Point it out or bring it closer. The dementia person will most often engage in a conversation with you about what is being seen. If sight is gone, you can be their eyes by vocalizing a detailed description of what you are seeing.

Rod had been a very successful pharmacist and loved the outdoors. During an antique car show we took him out to the parking lot to see the cars. At this time he was speaking very little but walked up to a 1932 Ford coupe, grabbed the handle, and said, "Let's take her for a spin!" The owner of the car, a woman, said, "Okay let's go". We loaded Rod into her car and she drove him up the block and back. What a thrill to watch his face just beaming!

The grandson of one of my patients loved to garden and would often bring in a beautiful bouquet. As I brought the flowers close, each person in turn would lean over to smell them and invariably would remark about the different colors. Many times the stimulation would lead one of them to reminisce about a long forgotten garden from the past. What treasured stories these were.

If your care receiver is restricted to being indoors, whether in a home or facility, bring as many delightful objects in as possible; flowers in the spring and summer, leaves in the fall, snow or rain in the winter. Rain? Yes, rain. Wear your raincoat in while the rain drops are still wet, show it and discuss the storm outside. Did she ever get caught in a storm? Did he enjoy splashing through mud puddles when he was young? Use your imagination. Be creative in bringing back those treasured memories. Provide the joy of the moment.

But, of course, not all stimuli are good! Television is so much a part of our everyday life that its influence is often overlooked. We get used to the drone of the TV which is often left on all day and all evening. *Very important!! Persons in the middle to late stages of a dementia should never be left to sit and watch non-selected television programs. Much of what is programmed is much too violent and stressful for a person with a dementia to handle.

An experience that really brought that point home for me was with an Alzheimer's afflicted, seventy-two year old man. Bert had been watching a violent movie just prior to being brought in to daycare. It is a fact that the memory impaired will often turn fantasy into reality, and in this case Bert was ready to hurt someone. He was very strong and it took a team of caregivers and activity staff over two hours to get him calmed down. Until this happened, Bert's wife had no idea that he may react this way from watching TV.

Even the daily news is, unfortunately, filled with grisly details that are not appropriate for dementia victims. Find other ways to fulfill the care receiver's desire to watch television or be very vigilant in monitoring what is being watched. It is difficult to stress the importance of this enough.

You may also notice that your patient likes to watch children's shows such as Sesame Street. This is fine, however, you still need to monitor the contents of the show and, perhaps, sit down and watch it with them. Many children's programs are just fine and very entertaining, but unfortunately, some are not at all appropriate.

The Sense of Touch

As dementia progresses and a person's abilities diminish, physical sensation may become one of the most important sources of communication and comfort.

Tactile items like tablecloths, towels, lace and satin seem to be very soothing to a person afflicted with a dementia. You may notice your care recipient gently rubbing a hand back and forth across the tablecloth after finishing a meal, or fingering the buttons on some article of clothing.

One of our dementia patients, Bob, loved to stand at the nurse's station. He would walk back and forth rubbing his hands on the smooth surface of the counter top. As I began to realize the joy that Bob got from this activity, I provided him with the added stimulus of a soft cloth. It was wonderful to watch him so absorbed in his activity and then to see his face simply light up when we praised him for helping us clean the counter.

Before Regina's dementia set in, she had owned several popular restaurants. She had lived a very busy life and her hands were always looking for something to do. She now spends hours helping out in the dining room by folding napkins. This activity allows Regina to feel a genuine sense of purpose and we always let her know how much she is helping us. Regina beams with pride when she hands us a pile of folded napkins.

Tactile articles can provide hours and hours of positive stimulation for your care receiver. Try to figure out what provides the pleasure of touch for that person. It could be anything but will no doubt be some fabric, hardware items or something that is reminiscent of the past. I have made several tactile boards for the benefit of my patients. One of them had a half dozen or so latches on it and Sam, a cabinet maker in the past, would spend hours every day, opening and closing those latches.

Hug and hold hands as often as your loved one will permit. Massage can be wonderful. If it is not too uncomfortable for you, rub his or her shoulders, feet and hands often. We now have come to understand more about the importance of massage for dementia patients. There are therapists who specialize in elder touch therapy. If it is affordable, seek one out—their service is incredibly valuable.

If you have the opportunity to go through the death process with your dementia person, sense of feeling may be the remaining sense. It is my belief, from what I have experienced, that soft touch makes passage easier. Your touch will let a loved one know that he or she is not alone.

CHAPTER EIGHT

Art Therapy

I remember well a wonderful man in his mid-eighties who was sincerely delighted to have the opportunity to paint. He told me he had always wanted to but never got the chance or had the time to paint because of his busy career as an engineer. He told me that painting with such beautiful colors was soothing to him. With each color he used he would tell me a story. He liked blue because it reminded him of the sky. He told me that when he was a young man he used to like to lie down in the grass of his fathers cow pasture and look up at the sky. He would pretend that he could travel any where in the world just by looking up at the sky and making such a wish. Other colors had other significant meanings to him, which we explored.

Art therapy can be both interesting and rewarding. You can offer different mediums such as paint, crayon, pencil and chalk. To eliminate confusion, it is best to limit the number of choices. If the care receiver does not participate immediately, try drawing a black line in the shape of a square, circle or rectangle; large permanent markers work well for this task. Involvement will usually follow immediately. You may also ask your "artist" to help you fill in the shape with some color. Limit the amount of color choice. If you notice that choosing is difficult, suggest use of his/her favorite color—everyone has a favorite color (Always use water based non-toxic paint.). Just because a person never had the opportunity or interest in art does not mean they will not enjoy an art project. Give it a try.

Art therapy can come from many different sources. Pictures cut from magazines can be used in collages. Do not hesitate to allow your care receiver to cut but be certain to provide blunt end paper scissors. Construction paper can be cut into different shapes and colors for a variety of projects, and coloring books and crayons can provide hours of fun activity.

Art therapy can play a very significant roll and for most patients becomes a valuable part of daily activities. It is very stimulating to the senses and yet, seems to be soothing to the nervous system.

If the things you try do not immediately generate interest, don't give up. It often takes time for interest to be stimulated again. When you accomplish that it can become something the person really looks forward to.

CHAPTER NINE

Providing Dignity

The most important aspect to remember, when dealing with any form of dementia, is to help the indisposed person to maintain dignity and self-esteem. Whether you are working with one person or a group your affirmation and reaffirmation needs to be continual. As your dementia person looses pieces of the former self, you may find yourself trying to pick those pieces up and place them back where they once were. Let it go.

Place your energy and emphasis on what is still there, and concentrate on those things. For example, there may come a time when the dementia person will not recognize you. Prepare yourself for this in advance. It may take a while to work through but you can do it. If your father becomes convinced that you are his brother, step into the role of the brother, tomorrow you may be his son again. The family members who can acknowledge the joy, love, and humor of each situation will gain the most from time spent with the afflicted loved one.

Continually remind the dementia person that he is loved, will always be loved, and that he will never be alone. One of the first things dementia tends to accomplish is to strip away one's feelings of self worth. Help your loved one to know dignity. It may well be the most important thing you can do to help that person live out their life in peace.

Conclusion

In reality we all live in the moment. Those of us who are not mentally restricted have the wonderful benefit of hoping and planning for the next moment, the next hour, the next day—and so on into the future. The theme of this booklet has been "the joy of the moment" because the right now is where the dementia patient lives, and where we must meet each of them in order to have meaningful interactions.

All of the things that I have shared with you I have some times referred to as therapy for the soul. That is because during all of the years of working with Alzheimer type afflictions my successes were measured, not by a paycheck at the end of the month, but by seeing old eyes that had become empty light up once again, and a stoic frown from forgotten dignity turn back into a grin. What I was able to do over the past years, and, hopefully, will continue to do is truly therapy, not only for the souls of my dementia patients, but for mine as well. Having the opportunity to interact with them in this way has been tremendously rewarding for me. I have learned that anytime I add joy into the life of another, that joy is returned many fold.

Know this and always keep it in mind. There is still a very real person in there who wants and deserves to live out their life with whatever joy and dignity we can help them to experience. Whatever your level of ability, whatever time you can dedicate, I hope you will make this your goal for the memory impaired person(s) in your family or facility: give them hugs and kisses, hold their hand, walk beside them. Show them the sunshine, rain and flowers. Tell them how much you love and care about them. Let them see your smile and allow them to give you one in return. Relax. Set aside a little time to enjoy the peace that your loving care can provide. Use your imagination to enrich a life in every way possible.

I have a genuine respect and admiration for all of you who are dedicating a part of your life, whether it be as a family member or as a clinician, to caring for the elderly dementia victim(s). It is my sincere hope that what I have shared in these pages will help you to give more joy, to receive more joy, and to experience the rewards. I urge you to let go and laugh as often as possible.

In the sunset of a loved one's life concentrate on the joy that can come about with each new sunrise. Give the demented person the light and let them become the star. You can make it happen.

Activities

Within the following pages you will be introduced to many forms of activity. These gentle exercises, fun games, old, songs, and familiar hymns have been specially selected to provide stimulation and/or initiate positive response in persons with memory impairment. I have used these activities continuously over the years and found them to be very effective as well as being a lot of fun. Of course, not all physical activities are appropriate for all patients. You will need to make that determination for your special patient.

The songs and hymns are in large print in order to be more readable. Please feel free to make copies so that each person in the singing group may see the words.

Enjoy!!

Daily
Stretch Routine

daily stretch routine

As part of your daily schedule, whether it is for one person or a group, I recommend an activity routine. The length of time for the program should be no more than one half hour. During this time you may read to the person or group from the newspaper for current events, share a reading from a book or pictures in a magazine, sing some songs and/or do some trivia. You may choose to read a daily devotion—maybe say the Lord's Prayer together. Include the pledge of allegiance to our American flag—the generation you are working with tends to be very patriotic. Try to sing at least three songs, singing is good exercise. It is very important to make this a routine—same time, same place, every day. In addition, it is so beneficial, at each meeting, to include an exercise routine as I have outlined below.

Save ten or fifteen minutes of your meeting for the following stretch routine. This routine will be executed from a sitting position. The leader will need to be in the middle while the group is seated around in a circle. This will allow the leader to demonstrate each stretch in front of each person as needed.

1) Have each person take his or her chin and place it on the chest—then back up again to normal position. Do not go upward much beyond normal position as this is can be hard on the neck. As you move around the circle you will be demonstrating the stretch. Repeat this neck stretch 6 times.

2)   Now, demonstrate, and have each person move an ear to the side until it touches the shoulder—then back up to normal position. Repeat this stretch 6 times.

3)   Now, move the other ear to the other shoulder, and repeat 6 times. Note that I do not ask for the right or left specifically because it does not really matter and could cause confusion. Just have them to start with either ear and then go to the other ear.

4)   Bring both shoulders upwards in a shrug position and back down to normal. Repeat 6 times. Watch for anyone who may be showing signs of fatigue or have difficulty with a particular stretch.

5)   Extend both hands out in front and shake them. Easy, now—not too fast. Hold the shake for 4 or 5 seconds.

6)   Demonstrate, and have them take a deep breath in through the nose and out through the mouth. Repeat a second time.

7)   Extend both hands out in front of you and cross them over the top of each other and back out. You will need to space a group out a bit so no one gets clobbered. Repeat 6-8 times.

8)   Next, bend your arms at the elbow with fists upwards towards your shoulders. Have them pretend they are holding a broom stick as they raise their fists up above the head. Again repeat 6-8 times.

9)   Extend your arms out in front again and wiggle your fingers as you pretend to play a piano. This stretch is good for arthritis in the hands. Hold the piano playing for several seconds.

10) Take another deep breath in through the nose and out through the mouth. Repeat again.

11) Now the upper body should be feeling like it has had some good stretching. We will now begin to work with the lower body.

12) While sitting extend one leg out in front of you and lift it up even with your chair, roll your ankle in one direction. Roll it in the same direction several times and then roll it back the opposite direction for the same amount of seconds. Put your foot down.

13) Now, do the same ankle roll with the opposite ankle. Hold for several seconds in one direction and then rotate it back the other way. Put your foot down.

14) Extend both feet out in front of you while lifting them off of the floor and flutter kick them. While kicking the feet get your arms in a swimming motion over your head and swim! Hold the swim motion for several seconds. Okay, now let's rest.

15) Take a deep breath in through your nose and out through your mouth. Repeat.

16) While sitting lift your feet one at a time off of the floor as though you are marching. Pretend to go for a walk, where will you walk today? Hold the walking motion for several seconds.

17) Now take another deep breath in through your nose and out through your mouth. Repeat one time.

At the close of your stretch you should be into the program for thirty minutes. If you have some extra time, you can always sing some more songs.

Thank everyone for coming to your meeting. You needed them to be there with you today and hope they can join you tomorrow at the same time.

Games

game instructions

Very important! Consult your dementia person's doctor if you question whether any activity may be unsafe for him or her.

You will note that my explanation of the different games include specific details on how to execute the different settings.

I recommend that all games be monitored. Watch any small pieces of game props so they are not placed in pockets or mouths.

All games and props should be stored away in a place that is not accessible to the patient(s).

Do not leave anything lying on the floor that could be tripped over.

In general, understand the limits of your game players, maintain common sense safety, and have fun.

Enjoy the Games!!

games

All facilities should be providing these types of games and activities for the well being of the patients. If you are a caregiver in your own home, you will realize similar benefits for your loved one. If the games are not playable with only two, adapt the ideas to make up your own version.

BALLOON TOSS

This simple game is my favorite and probably the most rewarding one you will ever use in a dementia situation. It will provide much laughter, exercise and sense of accomplishment. You should be using a large 16 inch inflated balloon. Tightly tied and safely stored these balloons, after inflation, can last for several weeks. Do not ask your person if they would like to play, just get their attention and give them a verbal cue like "here it comes David!"

In almost all cases, they will immediately raise their hand and hit it back to you. If they do not, cue them again with "please hit it back to me." Become as animated as possible, for every hit they give the balloon, reward them with positive remarks such as; "good job", "great hit", "good stretch", "great save"!

This game can be played in a family setting at home, a large group in a facility, or one on one. As the disease progresses this may be the last activity that your loved one will be capable of performing. Play it with a light spirit in your heart, and revel in the smiles around the room. Families will love playing this game together.

In large group settings your leader should know each person's name. If this is not possible, try to use name tags printed with their first names. Use their names to cue them that the balloon is coming their way. Remember to reward them as often as possible with positive uplifting remarks. Never patronize, even persons with dementia can always tell whether someone is sincere or not. You are working with an adult, always treat them with the dignity and respect that they deserve.

VOLLEYBALL

There are many elder sport catalogs where different games can be purchased. Most of them will carry a volleyball set. It will consist of two water filled stands, two posts and a net. If you do not have the room for or access to such a set, you can line up several chairs and tell your person to pretend that the line of chairs is the net.

Your players will remain seated in their chairs during the game. Do not allow them to get up and wander. You can place up to five chairs on each side of the net. Allow a few inches between chairs. Two helpers are needed to execute this game properly. The helpers are best placed standing behind the rows of chairs on each side of the net.

This is an active game. It is imperative that the staff members utilize their energy to maintain the game at its highest peak. To do this, be certain that every person is involved. If someone is not receiving the ball, arrange occasional hits directly to that person. Remain vocal and active, just as though you were involved in a championship game yourself! As in any game listed here, always make the players feel as though they are true champions—because they are! I have discovered that most of the people I have worked with were able to see bright yellow, pink or blue balloons the best. Dark colors like red and even orange are not as successful. I remember one dear lady who always watched the balloon long after her speech ability left her. When she could no longer play, she still loved to watch the balloon. Later I learned that she had played on a women's championship volleyball team! Calling out their name will help cue anyone who may not see the balloon coming their way. Use their names as often as possible during the game. Their efforts may be small but you will make them seem BIG!

BOWLING

After obtaining one of the many bowling games on the market today, begin by creating interest in the game. This can be one of the more strenuous games so not every one will be able to participate. But it can be fun for those who can. Try to set this game up in a highly visual room, where non players can see the activity. This can be a noisy game as the ball rolls across the floor. If you have someone who reacts unfavorably to noise, you might remove them to a quieter area. I prefer not to keep score on any game. That way everyone can be a winner!

Regardless of how poorly the ball rolls you must find a positive remark to make. The players must each be rewarded. Never ask them if they want to "try" to do something. Re-phrase the sentence to something such as we need you on our team; please come help us—I know you can do it.

In a group setting, some of your players may need to be aided by a helper as they throw the ball. This game is difficult for anyone who has difficulty ambulating and maintaining their balance.

GOLF

Yes, golf! A putting green can be purchased for under $30. Like bowling, not everyone can play, but they all like to watch and/or hear the activity. Start by setting it up in the middle of a common area. Be sure that there is ample room for anyone to walk around the game. Always monitor it after setting it up as it can be a tripping hazard.

Like bowling you will need to spot each person who plays. If the person cannot sink the ball after several attempts, allow them to move up the green until they get that hole in one. You will always refer to it as a "hole in one." Remember to give them the praise they deserve. Try to allow them to play as long as they would like. If they do not wish to stop playing, you might suggest they sit down and rest while someone else plays. Do not assume that they can judge how tired they become because usually they cannot.

This game usually requires at least two helpers, one to spot and one to catch and return the ball. With assistance, this game can be played from a wheel chair. The spotter will most likely need to help hold the club. This is a great game for families and friends to gather round and enjoy together.

If you question whether or not to attempt any activity, consult the patient's doctor.

PING PONG

There are many ping pong games on the market today. One of the best I have seen and used is a game I purchased through a children's party catalog for $6.00. It has become priceless to our staff. It consists of three plastic snap together net pieces, two snap on stands and two Nerf® balls. The Nerf® balls are quieter to use, and once you get used to them you will like them. The balls were colored yellow which made them easier to see.

For the wheelchair bound person you can remove the net, sit down and scoot the ball across the table to each other. The lady I created this setting for dubbed the game "old ladies ping pong." She loved to play!

I do not suggest that you allow two dementia victims to play each other. Again your helper must remain animated and praise the person at the end of the table. If you are in a facility, you can line up other interested persons in chairs on each side of the long table and ask them if they can help you catch the ball. You will be surprised at how they catch on and love to watch the ball and wait for their turn to keep the ball from hitting the floor.

BINGO

Regardless of the size of your group, bingo is always a big hit. The larger the group the more helpers you will need to assist in marking the numbers. You may need to cue your person when they need to yell bingo. Have a tray of gifts arranged on a tray and let them take their pick. Favorite snacks are always a hit. Like candy, both sugar and sugarless. I suggest only one card per player. You and any helpers will need to watch each person's card's for marked numbers and possible wins.

CROSSWORD PUZZLES

This is a setting that I created years ago in the facility where I worked. I used it in a large group setting but it can be adapted to home use with just two players. I would ask my player(s) to give me two words like "spring flowers". I would print the two words in large black print on a white board so the letters were vertical in two rows. Spring would print vertically on the left side of the board and flowers printed vertically on the right side of the board. Then, you will ask the player(s) to give you a word, any word, for each of the letters beginning with the letter "S." You may need to give some hints. Again not every one can join in, but most of them love to listen to the exchange.

When you have made words with each of the letters ask a helper to tell a story using all the words in the exact sequence they are listed. If you do not have a helper, you can tell the story your self or create a story with the help of your audience. The story telling is always enjoyed by the player(s) and audience alike.

PUZZLES

I recommend puzzles with no more than 100 pieces. This is easier to do in small sessions of one on one, or groups of no more than 3 or 4 people. Look for puzzles that have bright cheerful colors. One puzzle that never fails to please is a map of the United States. Puzzles are especially fun if children are around and would like to sit down and help find the pieces. It is an excellent way for children to learn how to interact in a dementia situation.

BOARD GAMES

Board games like Monopoly can be a challenge to play with someone with dementia. I have seen some success with Checkers and Yahtzee. If your loved one had a favorite board game, try it. It may work. Changing the rules to fit the abilities of the players is no crime and should be adopted. Kids are good at that so this becomes another excellent form of interaction for them. Whatever changes you make in rules must be done with dignity and respect for the person(s) involved in the game by asking for their consent.

CARD GAMES

Card games are generally best played in one to one or small group settings. Usually a person with dementia will not engage in cards unless they had played in previous years. If they did play, they will probably enjoy handling the cards. Don't hesitate to apply a little coaxing. Many times it takes some stimulus to get the mind going. I have seen some who always enjoyed playing solitaire. The game changed as their disease progressed, but they still enjoyed playing. At this point, the rules no longer matter.

Do not expect any memory impaired person to get up and go get the cards on their own. They will not do this. You must provide the stimulant by getting things started.

TRIVIA

To use the following favorite sayings, you the leader, will say the first part of the sentences and allow your person to respond with the answer which is underlined. If they do not respond, you may cue them with the answer. The more often you repeat them the more "wins" you can set up for your person. Many of these can lead into stories and reminisce sessions.

COMPLETE THESE SAYINGS

1. But for the grace of God, there go *(I).*

2. Every cloud has a (silver lining).

3. God helps them who help (themselves).

4. The pen is mightier than the (sword).

5. A bird in the hand is worth (two in the bush.)

6. I'll do it by hook or by (crook).

7. Rain, rain, go (away).

8. Come again another (day).

9. Nothing ventured, nothing (gained.)

10. I escaped by the skin of my (teeth.)

11. Time and tide wait for no (man).

12. One for the money, two for the (show).

13. Three to make ready, and four to (go).

14. Good things come to him who (waits.)

15. Never cry over spilled (milk.)

16. Too many cooks spoil (the broth.)

17. The first 100 years are the (hardest.)

18. This hits the nail on the (head.)

19. Don't look a gift horse in the (mouth).

20. Ali Baba and the forty (thieves).

21. Birds of a feather (flock together.)

22. Make hay while the sun (shines).

23. Rome was not built in a (day).

24. Honesty is the best (policy).

25. Live and let (live).

26. A watched pot never (boils).

27. Seven wonders of the (world).

28. A stitch in time saves (nine).

29. Out of sight, out of (mind).

30. Mad as a (March hare).

31. Love makes the world go (round).

32. One, two, buckle my (shoe).

33. Experience is the mother of (learning).

34. Sweet sixteen and never been (kissed).

35. Parting is such sweet (sorrow).

36. The moon is made of green (cheese).

37. Two is company, three's a (crowd).

38. Snug as a bug in a (rug).

39. Three wise (men).

40. A penny for your (thoughts).

41. Tale of two (cities).

42. Haste makes (waste).

43. Still waters run (deep).

44. A rolling stone gathers no (moss).

45. Wherever there is smoke there's (fire).

46. You can lead a horse to water but you can't make him (drink).

47. Never put off until tomorrow what you can do (today).

48. Home is where the (heart is).

49. Easy come, (easy go).

50. Possession is nine tenths of the (law).

51. I know on which side my bread is (buttered).

52. Music hath charms to soothe the (savage beast).

53. Eat, drink and be (merry).

54. It is better to be safe than (sorry).

55. Beauty is only (skin deep).

56. Don't count your chickens before they (hatch).

57. You can't have your cake and (eat it too).

58. When the cat's away, the mice will (play).

59. April showers bring (May flowers).

60. An apple a day keeps the (doctor away).

61. Practice makes (perfect).

62. Absence makes the heart grow (fonder).

63. Misery loves (company).

64. Love will find a (way).

65. One good turn deserves (another).

66. Paddle your own (canoe).

67. A group that sits around and talks a lot is shooting the (bull).

68. Someone who is anxious to go and wants to be first is an eager (beaver).

69. If someone really needs a bath we could say he is dirty as a (pig).

70. If someone is a little silly we say he has bats in his (belfry).

71. If someone has muscles and can lift heavy things we say he is strong as an (ox).

72. If you are nervous before you appear before a group of people, they say you have butterflies in your (stomach).

73. If the shoe fits, (wear it).

74. A fool and his money are soon (parted).

75. There's a sucker born every (minute).

76. The only thing we have to fear is (fear itself).

77. If at first you don't succeed, (try, try again).

78. I am the master of my fate, I am the captain of my (soul).

79. When we try to improve our self we say we are turning over a new (leaf).

80. Columbus sailed the ocean blue in (fourteen hundred ninety two).

81. Absence makes the heart grow (fonder).

82. Necessity is the mother of (invention).

83. Beauty is in the eye of the (beholder).

84. Someone who doesn't like to change his mind is stubborn as a (mule).

85. If you are very, very upset you might be mad as a (hornet).

86. If you are in bad situation and plan to get in another bad situation you are getting out of the frying pan and into the (fire.)

87. If a gal is really cute you might say she is quite a (dish).

88. If you feel good with a friend you say they are comfortable as an old (shoe).

89. If someone grows up in a wealthy family you say they are born with a silver (spoon in their mouth).

90. If children are around, you might not want to tell a secret because little pitchers (have big ears).

91. If you know someone did something wrong and you tell on them you are a (stool pigeon).

92. If you take someone for granted and are always "walking on them", you are treating them like a (doormat).

93. When a group of people get together because they have a lot in common, it is said, birds of a feather (flock together).

94. When a girl has a pretty complexion we could say her complexion is like peaches and (cream).

95. When someone is always grouchy, we say they have a chip on their (shoulder).

96. If you are doing a real good job of dancing you are cutting a (rug).

97. To leave a situation undisturbed is to "let sleeping dogs (lie)".

98. A person who refuses to learn a new way of doing something is described by the saying—you can't teach an old dog (new tricks).

99. March comes in like a lion and goes out like a (lamb).

100. Everybody talks about the weather but nobody (does anything about it.)

101. The stockings were hung by the chimney with care, in hopes that (St. Nicholas soon would be there.)

102. Listen, my children, and you shall hear, of the midnight ride of (Paul Revere).

103. I think that I shall never see a poem as lovely as a (tree).

104. Laugh and the world laughs with you, cry and you (cry alone).

105. To be or not to be, that is the (question).

106. But as for me, give me liberty (or give me death).

107. Mid pleasures and palaces though we may roam, be it ever so humble, there's no place like (home).

108. Man's work lasts till set of sun but woman's work (is never done).

109. The hand that rocks the cradle is the hand that (rules the world).

110. It is easier for a camel to go through the eye of a needle, than a rich man to enter the (kingdom of heaven).

111. When something pleasant happens to a person who has been having bad luck we say every dog (has his day).

112. If you look for something in the wrong place it is said you are barking up the (wrong tree).

Songs and Hymns

Songs

<u>*YOU ARE MY SUNSHINE*</u>

YOU ARE MY SUNSHINE
MY ONLY SUNSHINE
YOU MAKE ME HAPPY
WHEN SKIES ARE GREY

YOU'LL NEVER KNOW DEAR
HOW MUCH I LOVE YOU
PLEASE DON'T TAKE
MY SUNSHINE AWAY

THE OTHER NIGHT DEAR
AS I LAY SLEEPING
I DREAMED I HELD YOU
IN MY ARMS

WHEN I AWOKE DEAR
I WAS MISTAKEN
SO I HUNG MY HEAD
AND CRIED

YOU ARE MY SUNSHINE
MY ONLY SUNSHINE

YOU MAKE ME HAPPY
WHEN SKIES ARE GREY

YOU'LL NEVER KNOW DEAR
HOW MUCH I LOVE YOU
PLEASE DON'T TAKE MY
SUNSHINE AWAY

<u>*MY BONNIE LIES OVER THE OCEAN*</u>

MY BONNIE LIES OVER THE OCEAN
MY BONNIE LIES OVER THE SEA
MY BONNIE LIES OVER THE OCEAN
OH BRING BACK MY BONNIE TO ME.

BRING BACK, BRING BACK
OH BRING BACK MY BONNIE TO ME, TO ME.

BRING BACK, BRING BACK
OH BRING BACK MY BONNIE TO ME.

MY BONNIE LIES OVER THE OCEAN
MY BONNIE LIES OVER THE SEA
MY BONNIE LIES OVER THE OCEAN
OH BRING BACK MY BONNIE TO ME.

BRING BACK, BRING BACK
OH BRING BACK MY BONNIE TO ME, TO ME.

MY BONNIE LIES OVER THE OCEAN
MY BONNIE LIES OVER THE SEA
MY BONNIE LIES OVER THE OCEAN
OH BRING BACK MY BONNIE TO ME.

HOME ON THE RANGE

OH, GIVE ME A HOME
WHERE THE BUFFALO ROAM
WHERE THE DEER AND THE ANTELOPE PLAY.

WHERE SELDOM IS HEARD
A DISCOURAGING WORD
AND THE SKIES ARE NOT CLOUDY ALL DAY.

HOME, HOME ON THE RANGE WHERE THE DEER
AND THE ANTELOPE PLAY.

WHERE SELDOM IS HEARD A DISCOURAGING
WORD AND THE SKIES
ARE NOT CLOUDY ALL DAY.

IN THE GOOD OLD SUMMER TIME
George Evans & Ren Shields 1902

IN THE GOOD OLD SUMMERTIME,
IN THE GOOD OLD SUMMERTIME.
STROLLING DOWN THE SHADY LANE
WITH YOUR BABY MINE.

YOU HOLD HER HAND AND SHE HOLDS
YOURS, AND THAT'S A VERY GOOD SIGN,
THAT SHE'S YOUR TOOTSIE WOOTSIE
IN THE GOOD OLD SUMMERTIME.

MY WILD IRISH ROSE
Chauncy Olcott 1898

MY WILD IRISH ROSE
THE SWEETEST FLOWER THAT GROWS,
YOU MAY SEARCH EVERYWHERE,
BUT NONE CAN COMPARE,
WITH MY WILD IRISH ROSE.

MY WILD IRISH ROSE,
THE DEAREST FLOWER THAT GROWS
AND SOMEDAY FOR MY SAKE,
SHE MAY LET ME TAKE,
THE BLOOM FROM MY WILD IRISH ROSE.

BICYCLE BUILT FOR TWO

DAISY, DAISY,
GIVE ME YOUR ANSWER DO!

I'M HALF CRAZY,
ALL FOR THE LOVE OF YOU!

IT WON'T BE A STYLISH MARRIAGE,
I CAN'T AFFORD A CARRIAGE,

BUT YOU'LL LOOK SWEET,
UPON THE SEAT,

OF A BICYCLE BUILT FOR TWO!

OLD MACDONALD HAD A FARM

OLD MAC DONALD HAD A FARM
E-I-E-I-O!
AND ON HIS FARM HE HAD SOME CHICKS
E-I-E-I-O
WITH A CHICK, CHICK, HERE AND A
CHICK, CHICK, THERE,
HERE A CHICK, THERE A CHICK,
EVERYWHERE A CHICK, CHICK.

OLD MAC DONALD HAD A FARM
E-I-E-I-O
AND ON HIS FARM HE HAD SOME DUCKS
E-I-E-I-O
WITH A QUACK, QUACK, HERE AND A
QUACK, QUACK THERE,
HERE A QUACK, THERE A QUACK,
EVERYWHERE A QUACK, QUACK.

OLD MACDONALD HAD A FARM
E-I-E-I-O!

OH SUSANNA
Foster 1848

I'VE COME FROM ALABAMA
WITH MY BANJO ON MY KNEE.
I'M GOIN' TO LOUISANA,
MY TRUE LOVE FOR TO SEE.

IT RAINED ALL NIGHT,
THE DAY I LEFT,
THE WEATHER IT WAS DRY,
THE SUN SO HOT I FROZE TO DEATH,
SUSANNA, DON'T YOU CRY.

OH, SUSANNA
OH DON'T YOU CRY FOR ME,
I'VE COME FROM ALABAMA,
WITH MY BANJO ON MY KNEE.

OH, SUSANNA
OH, DON'T YOU CRY FOR ME,
I'VE COME FROM ALABAMA
WITH MY BANJO ON MY KNEE.

WHERE HAS MY LITTLE DOG GONE?

OH WHERE, OH WHERE
HAS MY LITTLE DOG GONE?

OH WHERE, OH WHERE CAN HE BE?

WITH HIS EARS CUT SHORT
AND HIS TAIL CUT LONG
OH WHERE, OH WHERE CAN HE BE?

SAILING

SAILING, SAILING
OVER THE BOUNDING MAIN,
FOR MANY A STORMY WIND SHALL BLOW "ERE
JACK COMES HOME AGAIN.

SAILING, SAILING
OVER THE BOUNDING MAIN,
FOR MANY A STORMY WIND SHALL BLOW 'ERE
JACK COMES HOME AGAIN.

I'VE BEEN WORKING ON THE RAILROAD

I'VE BEEN WORKING ON THE RAILROAD,
ALL THE LIVE LONG DAY

I'VE BEEN WORKING ON THE RAILROAD,
JUST TO PASS THE TIME AWAY

CAN'T YOU HEAR THE WHISTLE
BLOWING?

RISE UP SO EARLY IN THE MORN'
CAN'T YOU HEAR THE CAPTAIN
SHOUTING?

"DINAH, BLOW YOUR HORN!"

DINAH, WON'T YOU BLOW
DINAH WON'T YOU BLOW
DINAH, WON'T YOU BLOW YOUR HORN?

SOMEONE'S IN THE KITCHEN WITH DINAH,
SOMEONE'S IN THE KITCHEN I KNOW-OW-OW.
SOMEONE'S IN THE KITCHEN WITH DINAH-
STRUMMIN ON THE OLD BANJO!

THE CAISSONS GO ROLLING ALONG
Edmund L. Gruber 1908

OVER HILL, OVER DALE WE WILL HIT
THE DUSTY TRAIL
AND THOSE CAISSONS GO ROLLING ALONG.
IN AND OUT, HEAR THEM SHOUT,
"COUNTER MARCH AND LEFT ABOUT,"
AND THOSE CAISSONS GO ROLLING ALONG.

AND IT'S HI-HI-HEE
IN THE FIELD ARTILLERY
SO SHOUT OUT YOUR NUMBERS
LOUD AND STRONG (2, 3)
FOR WHERE EVER YOU GO
YOU WILL ALWAYS KNOW
THAT THOSE CAISSONS
GO ROLLING ALONG.

Hymns

AMERICA, THE BEAUTIFUL

Katharine Lee Bates   Samuel A. Ward

O BEAUTIFUL FOR SPACIOUS SKIES, FOR AMBER WAVES OF GRAIN, FOR PURPLE MOUNTAIN MAJESTIES ABOVE THE FRUITED PLAIN!

AMERICA! AMERICA! GOD SHED HIS GRACE ON THEE, AND CROWN THY GOOD WITH BROTHER-HOOD FROM SEA TO SHINING SEA!

O BEAUTIFUL FOR HEROES PROVED IN LIBERAT-ING STRIFE, WHO MORE THAN SELF THEIR COUN-TRY LOVED, AND MERCY MORE THAN LIFE! AMERICA! AMERICA! MAY GOD THY GOLD REFINE 'TIL ALL SUCCESS BE NOBLENESS, AND EVERY GAIN DIVINE!

O BEAUTIFUL FOR PATIRIOT DREAM THAT SEES BEYOND THE YEARS, THINE ALABASTER CITIES GLEAM, UNDIMMED BY HUMAN TEARS!

AMERICA! AMERICA! GOD SHED HIS GRACE ON THEE, AND CROWN THY GOOD WITH BROTHERHOOD FROM SEA TO SHINING SEA!

BRINGING IN THE SHEAVES

Knowles Shaw   George A. Minor

SOWING IN THE MORNING, SOWING SEEDS OF KINDNESS, SOWING IN THE NOONTIDE AND THE DEWY EVE; WAITING FOR THE HARVEST AND THE TIME OF REAPING. WE SHALL COME REJOICING BRINGING IN THE SHEAVES.

BRINGING IN THE SHEAVES, BRINGING IN THE SHEAVES. WE SHALL COME REJOICING, BRINGING IN THE SHEAVES. BRINGING IN THE SHEAVES, BRINGING IN THE SHEAVES. WE SHALL COME REJOICING, BRINGING IN THE SHEAVES.

SOWING IN THE SUNSHINE, SOWING IN THE SHADOWS, FEARING NEITHER CLOUDS NOR WINTER'S CHILLING BREEZE; BY AND BY THE HARVEST AND LABOR ENDED, WE SHALL COME REJOICING, BRINGING IN THE SHEAVES.

AT CALVARY

Wm. R. Newell   Daniel B. Towner

YEARS I SPENT IN VANITY AND PRIDE, CARING NOT MY LORD WAS CRUCIFIED, KNOWING NOT IT WAS FOR ME HE DIED, ON CALVARY.

MERCY THERE WAS GREAT, AND GRACE WAS FREE; PARDON THERE WAS MULTIPLIED TO ME; THERE MY BURDENED SOUL FOUND LIBERTY, AT CALVARY

NOW I'VE GIVEN TO JESUS EVERYTHING; NOW I GLADLY OWN HIM AS MY KING; NOW MY RAP-TURED SOUL CAN ONLY SING OF CALVERY

MERCY THERE WAS GREAT, AND GRACE WAS FREE; PARDON THERE WAS MULTIPLIED TO ME; THERE MY BURDENED SOUL FOUND LIBERTY, AT CALVARY!

WHEN THE ROLL IS CALLED

James M. Black   James M. Black

WHEN THE TRUMPET OF THE LORD SHALL SOUND AND TIME SHALL BE NO MORE, AND THE MORNING BREAKS ETERNAL, BRIGHT AND FAIR; WHEN THE SAVED OF EARTH SHALL GATHER OVER ON THE OTHER SHORE, AND THE ROLL IS CALLED UP YONDER, I'LL BE THERE.

WHEN THE ROLL, IS CALLE D UP YONDER, WHEN THE ROLL, IS CALLED UP YONDER, WHEN THE ROLL, IS CALLED UP YONDER, WHEN THE ROLL IS CALLED UP YONDER, I'LL BE THERE

ON THAT BRIGHT AND CLOUDLESS MORNING WHEN THE DEAD IN CHRIST SHALL RISE, AND THE GLORY OF HIS RESURRECTION SHARE; WHEN HIS CHOSEN ONES SHALL GATHER TO THEIR HOME BEYOND THE SKIES, AND THE ROLL IS CALLED UP YONDER, I'LL BE THERE.

WHAT A FRIEND WE HAVE IN JESUS

Joseph Scriven   Charles C. Converse

WHAT A FRIEND WE HAVE IN JESUS, ALL OUR SINS
AND GRIEFS TO BEAR, WHAT A PRIVILEGE TO
CARRY EVERYTHING TO
GOD IN PRAYER.

OH, WHAT PEACE WE OFTEN FORFEIT, OH, WHAT
NEEDLESS PAIN WE BEAR.
ALL BECAUSE WE DO NOT CARRY EVERYTHING TO
GOD IN PRAYER.

ARE WE WEAK AND HEAVY LADEN, CUMBERED
WITH A LOAD OF CARE? PRECIOUS SAVIOUR, STILL
OUR REFUGE TAKE IT TO THE LORD IN PRAYER.

DO THY FRIENDS DESPISE, FORSAKE THEE? TAKE
IT TO THE LORD IN PRAYER.
IN HIS ARMS HE'LL TAKE AND SHIELD THEE;
THOU WILT FIND A SOLACE THERE.

MY COUNTRY 'TIS OF THEE

S.F. Smith   Henry Carey

MY COUNTRY, 'TIS OF THEE, SWEET LAND OF LIB-ERTY, OF THEE I SING;
LAND WHERE MY FATHERS DIED, LAND OF THE PILGRIMS' PRIDE, FROM EVERY MOUNTAINSIDE, LET FREEDOM RING.

MY NATIVE COUNTRY, THEE, LAND OF THE NOBLE FREE, THY NAME I LOVE.
I LOVE THY ROCKS AND RILLS, THY WOODS AND TEMPLED HILLS; MY HEART WITH RAPTURE THRILLS LIKE THAT ABOVE.

OUR FATHERS' GOD, TO THEE, AUTHOR OF LIB-ERTY, TO THEE WE SING;
LONG MAY OUR LAND BE BRIGHT WITH FREE-DOM'S HOLY LIGHT; PROTECT US BY THY MIGHT, GREAT GOD, OUR KING.

HOW GREAT THOU ART!

Stuart K. Hine

O LORD MY GOD, WHEN I IN AWESOME WONDER CONSIDER ALL THE WORKS THY HANDS HATH MADE; I SEE THE STARS, I HEAR THE MIGHTY THUNDER, THY POW'R THROUGHOUT THE UNIVERSE DISPLAYED.

THEN SINGS MY SOUL, MY SAVIOR GOD, TO THEE;
HOW GREAT THOU ART, HOW GREAT THOU ART!
THEN SINGS MY SOUL, MY SAVIOR GOD, TO THEE;
HOW GREAT THOU ART, HOW GREAT THOU ART!

AND WHEN I THINK THAT GOD, HIS SON NOT SPARING, SENT HIM TO DIE, I SCARCE CAN TAKE IT IN, THAT ON THE CROSS, MY BURDEN GLADLY BEARING, HE BLED AND DIED TO TAKE AWAY MY SIN!

THEN SINGS MY SOUL, MY SAVIOR GOD, TO THEE;
HOW GREAT THOU ART, HOW GREAT THOU ART!
THEN SINGS MY SOUL, MY SAVIOR GOD, TO THEE;
HOW GREAT THOU ART, HOW GREAT THOU ART!

JESUS LOVES ME

Anna B. Warner   William B. Bradbury

JESUS LOVES ME, THIS I KNOW, FOR THE BIBLE
TELLS ME SO.
LITTLE ONES TO HIM BELONG, THEY ARE WEAK
BUT HE IS STRONG.

YES, JESUS LOVES ME. YES, JESUS LOVES ME. YES,
JESUS LOVES ME. THE BIBLE TELLS ME SO.

JESUS LOVES ME, HE WHO DIED, HEAVEN'S GATES
TO OPEN WIDE.
HE WILL WASH AWAY MY SIN, LET HIS LITTLE
CHILD COME IN.

YES, JESUS LOVES ME. YES, JESUS LOVES ME. YES,
JESUS LOVES ME. THE BIBLE TELLS ME SO.

JESUS, TAKE THIS HEART OF MINE. MAKE IT PURE
AND WHOLLY THINE. THOU HAST BLED AND DIED
FOR ME. I WILL HENCEFORTH LIVE FOR THEE.

YES, JESUS LOVES ME. YES, JESUS LOVES ME. YES,
JESUS LOVES ME. THE BIBLE TELLS ME SO.

ONWARD CHRISTIAN SOLDIERS

Sabine Baring-Gould   Arthur Sullivan

ONWARD, CHRISTIAN SOLDIERS, MARCHING AS TO WAR, WITH THE CROSS OF JESUS GOING ON BEFORE. CHRIST, THE ROYAL MASTER, LEADS AGAINST THE FOE FORWARD INTO BATTLE, SEE HIS BANNERS GO.

ONWARD, CHRISTIAN SOLDIERS, MARCHING AS TO WAR, WITH THE CROSS OF JESUS GOING ON BEFORE.

ONWARD, THEN YE PEOPLE. JOIN OUR HAPPY THRONG, BLEND WITH OURS YOUR VOICES IN THE TRIUMPH SONG. GLORY, LAUD, AND HONOR UNTO CHRIST, THE KING; THIS THRO' COUNT-LESS AGES, MEN AND ANGELS SING.

ONWARD, CHRISTIAN SOLDIERS, MARCHING AS TO WAR, WITH THE CROSS OF JESUS GOING ON BEFORE!

IN THE GARDEN

C.A.M.   C. Austin Miles

I COME TO THE GARDEN ALONE, WHILE THE DEW IS STILL ON THE ROSES; AND THE VOICE I HEAR FALLING ON MY EAR, THE SON OF GOD DISCLOSES.

AND HE WALKS WITH ME, AND HE TALKS WITH ME, AND HE TELLS ME I AM HIS OWN, AND THE JOY WE SHARE AS WE TARRY THERE, NONE OTHER HAS EVER KNOWN.

HE SPEAKS, AND THE SOUND OF HIS VOICE IS SO SWEET THE BIRDS HUSH THEIR SINGING; AND THE MELODY THAT HE GAVE TO ME WITHIN MY HEART IS RINGING.

AND HE WALKS WITH ME AND HE TALKS WITH ME, AND HE TELLS ME I AM HIS OWN, AND THE JOY WE SHARE AS WE TARRY THERE, NONE OTHER HAS EVER KNOWN.

ROCK OF AGES

Augustus M. Toplady   Thomas Hastings

ROCK OF AGES, CLEFT FOR ME, LET ME HIDE MYSELF IN THEE. LET THE WATER AND THE BLOOD, FROM THY WOUNDED SIDE WHICH FLOWED, BE OF SIN THE DOUBLE CURE, SAVE FROM WRATH AND MAKE ME PURE.

COULD MY TEARS FOREVER FLOW, COULD MY ZEAL NO LANGUOR KNOW. THESE FOR SIN COULD NOT ATONE; THOU MUST SAVE AND THOU ALONE, IN MY HAND NO PRICE I BRING; SIMPLY TO THY CROSS I CLING.

WHILE I DRAW THIS FLEETING BREATH, WHEN MY EYES SHALL CLOSE IN DEATH, WHEN I RISE TO WORLDS UNKNOWN, AND BEHOLD THEE ON THY THRONE. ROCK OF AGES CLEFT FOR ME, LET ME HIDE MYSELF IN THEE.

BATTLE HYMN OF THE REPUBLIC

Julis Ward Howe   American Melody

MINE EYES HAVE SEEN THE GLORY OF THE COM-
ING OF THE LORD, HE IS TRAMPLING OUT THE
VINTAGE WHERE THE GRAPES OF WRATH ARE
STORED; HE HATH LOOSED THE FATEFUL LIGHT-
NING OF HIS TERRIBLE SWIFT SWORD, HIS TRUTH
IS MARCHING ON.

GLORY! GLORY! HALLELUJAH! GLORY! GLORY! HAL-
LELUJAH! GLORY! GLORY! HALLELUJAH! HIS
TRUTH IS MARCHING ON.

HE HAS SOUNDED FORTH THE TRUMPET THAT
SHALL NEVER CALL RETREAT, HE IS SIFTING OUT
THE HEARTS OF MEN BEFORE HIS JUDGMENT
SEAT; O BE SWIFT, MY SOUL, TO ANSWER HIM, BE
JUBILANT, MY FEET! OUR GOD IS MARCHING ON.

IN THE BEAUTY OF THE LILIES CHRIST WAS BORN
ACROSS THE SEA, WITH A GLORY IN HIS BOSOM
THAT TRANSFIGURES YOU AND ME;
AS HE DIED TO MAKE MEN HOLY LET US LIVE TO
MAKE MEN FREE! WHILE GOD IS MARCHING ON.

Joy Notes

Special moments with_____

Recorded by_____

Joy Notes

Joy Notes

Joy Notes

Joy Notes

Joy Notes

Joy Notes

Joy Notes

Joy Notes

Joy Notes

Joy Notes

Joy Notes

Joy Notes

Joy Notes

<u>Joy Notes</u>

0-595-25748-8

Printed in the United States
19895LVS00007B/121-147